Issues
Of
Ejaculation
Resolved

Refuge Victor

Table of content

Chapter one

Ejaculation

Discharge is the point at which you discharge semen (cum) from your penis. It, for the most part, transpires when an individual with a penis arrives athe t climax (sexual peak), however, it can likewise occur without climax.

What is discharge?
Discharge is the point at which a tacky fluid (semen or cum) emerges from your penis. It most frequently occurs after a climax (a sexual delivery), however can likewise occur without a climax.

What happens when you are discharged?
Your sensory system controls discharge. Nerves that go from your regenerative framework to parts of your spinal string force semen out of your penis when sexual energy arrives at a fundamentally undeniable level.

Discharge has two stages: emanation and removal.

Emanation stage: In the principal stage, sperm moves to your prostate from your balls and blends in with liquid to make semen. Your vas deferens (the cylinders that store and transport semen from your testiclagreement tress the semen toward the foundation of your penis.

Ejection stage: In the subsequent stage, muscles at the foundation of your penis contract each second and power or shoot the semen out of your penis in a few sprays.

How frequently should a man be discharged is certainly not a limited sum for how frequently you ought to be discharged. Research shows discharge has numerous medical advantages like diminishing an individual's gamble for prostate disease. Yet, there isn't proof that not discharging causes medical conditions. As the outcomes are uncertain, it's ideal to have a conversation with your medical care supplier if you have worries about how much of the time you discharge.

What occurs assuming that you hold discharge in?

Holding discharge in or preventing yourself from discharge when you arrive at the place of climax isn't genuinely imaginable, as it's a programmed reaction. On the off chance that you're irritated by an untimely discharge, converse with a medical services supplier, as there might be therapies to assist you with postponing discharge.

At what age does discharge start?

Discharge normally begins when an individual starts creating sperm around the time of pubescence. Adolescence occurs at various times for various individuals. By and large, individuals start pubescence somewhere in the range of 10 and 12 years of age. This implies an individual might discharge interestingly inside this age range. An individual for the most part discharges interestfully during a "wet dream" or after jerking off. Once more, the specific timing shifts, however, you can anticipate that an individual should have the option to discharge in the span of a while to an extended period of pubescence starting. You can in any case jerk off without discharge. Numerous youngsters experience delight and jerk off before they can discharge.

What are the most widely recognized discharge issues?
There are three fundamental discharge issues you might have

Untimely discharge: When the discharge charge is sooner than you or your accomplice would like. This timing can change contingent upon the individual, yet all the same, it's considered normal.

Deferred discharge: It takes a ton of sexual feeling for you to discharge. Certain individuals don't discharge by any means. For instance, somebody who needs sex for 45 minutes before they discharge might be encountering deferred discharge.
Retrograde discharge: A condition that makes semen stream in reverse into your urethra and bladder rather than out of your penis.

Converse with your medical services supplier on the off chance that you assume you disapprove of discharge. There are treatment choices to help you.

Discharge is the point at which you discharge semen from your penis. It most frequently happens during the sexual peak or climax. There are a few issues related to discharge. Contact a medical care supplier except you generally disapprove of discharge.

Chapter two

Premature Ejaculation

Untimely discharge happens when a man has a climax and discharges prior during inteintercostalor his accomplice would like. It's a typical issue, influencing 30% to 40% of men. Causes incorporate actual issues, substance uneven characters, and profound/mental variables. Medicines incorporate learning procedures to postpone discharge.

What is an untimely discharge?

Untimely discharge is a kind of sexual brokenness that happens when a man has a climax and deals delivery charges) semen sooner than he or his accomplice would like. It frequently occurs previously or not long after infiltration during intercourse. Untimely discharge can be a disappointing encounter for both you and your sexual accomplice and makes your sexual experiences less pleasant. Notwithstanding, fortunately, it's, normally fixable!

How normal is untimely discharge?

Somewhere in the range of 30% and 40% of men experience untimely discharge eventually in their life. As per the American Urological Affiliation, untimely discharge is the most well-known sort of sexual brokenness in men. Around one of every five men between the ages of 18 and 59 report frequencies of untimely discharge.

What time span therapeutically characterizes a man's discharge as untimely?

Albeit the meaning of untimely discharge shifts, the American Urological Affiliation characterizes discharge as "untimely" if it happens sooner than wanted, either previously or not long after the entrance, making trouble possibly one or the two accomplices. The American Mental Affiliation characterizes three degrees of seriousness (gentle, moderate, extreme), in light of time to discharge, with gentle being under one moment. Whenever squeezed for some time, many specialists would characterize rashness as discharge in nothing less than a moment of starting intercourse. Notwithstanding proficient suppositions, your sentiments regarding what is untimely are likewise thought of.

What causes untimely discharge?
Physical, compound, and profound/mental variables cause untimely discharge.

Physical and substance issues include:

- A fundamental erectile brokenness finding.
- A hormonal issue with oxytocin levels, which plays a part in sexual capability in men. Other chemical levels that assume a part in sexual capability incorporate luteinizing chemical (LH), prolactin, and thyroid-animating chemical (TSH)
- Low serotonin or dopamine levels are synthetic substances in the mind that are engaged with sexual longing and energy.
- A penis that is additionally delicate to excitement.

Profound or mental causes include:

Execution uneasiness. This could be because of the anxiety of being with another accomplice, the uneasiness of engaging in sexual relations again after an extensive stretch of restraint, the absence of certainty, responsibility, being excessively energized or invigorated, or different reasons.
- Stress.
- Relationship issues.
- Discouragement.

Are there different side effects of untimely discharge?
No. The main side effect of untimely discharge is the actual condition.

How are the reasons for untimely discharge analyzed?

If you have regular untimely discharges, or on the other hand on the off chance that untimely discharge is causing you tension or sorrow and influencing your relationship, plan to see a urologist.

Your urologist will start a test by getting some information about your sexual encounters. You will probably be inquired:

- How long have you had this issue?
- Under what conditions does it work out?
- How frequently does it work out?
- Does untimely discharge occur at each sexual endeavor?
- Does it occur with all accomplices?
- Does untimely discharge happen when you jerk off?
- Do you experience difficulty keeping an erection?

While the inquiries are private, you should answer your urologist genuinely so they can best analyze the wellspring of your concern.

Your urologist will likewise get some information about some other ailments you might have and any meds including non-prescription meds, enhancements, and natural items you are taking. You will likewise get some information about any liquor and unlawful medication use.

- Are lab tests expected to analyze untimely discharge?

Lab tests are normally not required except if your medical services supplier thinks that a hidden medical condition is adding to the issue.

How is untimely discharge treated?

There are various medicine choices for untimely discharge contingent upon the reason. These incorporate social treatment, advising, and meds. Most reasons for untimely discharge are normally treated first with conduct treatment as well as directed to assist with profound worries, execution uneasiness, or stressors that might contribute. Frequently more than one treatment approach might be attempted simultaneously.

Conduct treatment

Conduct treatment includes attempting various strategies to postpone your climax. It will probably show you how to control your body and your sentiments. Strategies include:

Begin and stop: With this method, you or your accomplice animates your penis near the mark of climax and then, at that point, stops the feeling for around 30 seconds until you recapture control of your reaction. Rehash this "begin and stop" move three or multiple times before permitting yourself to climax. Keep rehearsing this technique until you have acquired great control.

Crush treatment: With this procedure, you or your accomplice animates your penis near the mark of climax then, at that point, delicately presses the top of your penis for around 30 seconds so you start to lose your erection. Rehash this strategy a couple of times before permitting yourself to climax. Keep rehearsing this procedure until you have acquired control in postponing your climax.

Occupied thinking: With this method, the thought is to concentrate on standard nonsexual things while you're physically invigorated. Naming successions are an effective method for concentrating. For instance, imagine naming every one of the organizations you give your drive to the rec center, naming every one of the players in your number one games group, or naming every one of the items on the passageways of your #1 store.

Guiding
If the reason for your untimely discharge is mental, personal, or because of relationship issues - because of execution nervousness, melancholy,

stress, responsibility, or a pained relationship - look for the assistance of a clinician, specialist, couples specialist, or sex specialist. Your urologist can assist with guiding you to this well-being.

Drugs
A few sorts of prescriptions might be attempted.

Antidepressants, particularly specific serotonin reuptake inhibitors like citalopram (Celexa®), escitalopram (Lexapro®), fluoxetine (Prozac®), paroxetine (Paxil®), and sertraline (Zoloft®) or the tricyclic stimulant clomipramine (Anafranil®), can assist with postponing untimely discharge. This is an "off-mark" use (not endorsed by the Food and Medication Organization for this utilization). Make certain to talk about the symptoms of this prescription with your urologist to be certain it's fitting for you.

Sedative (desensitizing) creams and splashes applied to the head and shaft of the penis are one more drug choice to defer discharge. The sedative cream or shower is applied to the penis, retained for 10 to 30 minutes or until you feel less awareness in your penis. It means a lot to wash your penis before sex to forestall deadness to your accomplice's vagina or loss of your erection.

Erectile brokenness prescriptions, which incorporate sildenafil (Viagra®), tadalafil (Cialis®), vardenafil (Levitra®), and Avanafil (Stendra®), have likewise been utilized to treat untimely discharge, especially in men with fundamental erectile brokenness.

Are lab tests expected to conclude untimely discharge?
Lab tests are typically not required except if your medical care supplier thinks that a hidden medical condition is adding to the issue.

Might I at any point forestall untimely discharge?
Indeed, you probably can! By following the methods depicted in this article to postpone discharge, taking any endorsed drugs, and looking for

guidance if necessary, untimely discharge can turn into an issue of your past.

Standpoint/Anticipation

What result could I at any point expect assuming that I have an untimely discharge?

There are a few treatment techniques that can assist with forestalling untimely discharge. By including your accomplice and seeing the proper medical services experts - a urologist for introductory evaluation in addition to other medical services experts (clinicians, specialists, guides) depending on the situation for fundamental contributing issues, you can probably control your discharge and partake in your sexual coexistence by and by.

Could wearing a condom assist with untimely discharge?

Indeed. Wearing a condom can diminish aversion to your penis and assist with postponing discharge.

Is untimely discharge destructive or an indication of a clinical issue?

The untimely discharge itself isn't destructive however other medical issues might add to the advancement of untimely discharge. These medical issues include:

Erectile brokenness (man can't keep a firm erection for intercourse).

Persistent pelvic torment condition (long haul torment and squeezing in the pelvic region in addition to long haul urinary parcel side effects and sexual brokenness).

- Thyroid problems.
- Sporting medication use.

What's the distinction between erectile brokenness and untimely discharge?

On the off chance that you have erectile brokenness, you can't accomplish or keep up with your erection. Assuming that you have an untimely discharge, you have an erection however you arrive at the climax and discharge sooner than you or your accomplice would have loved.

Be that as it may, erectile brokenness can prompt the advancement of untimely discharge. This happens when a man knows his capacity to support an erection is poor, so he fosters the propensity for discharging not long after erection before he loses his erection.

Due to this association between these two circumstances, your urology will need to sort out whether or not you have erectile brokenness and, provided that this is true, treat that first.

Will drinking liquor assist with deferring discharge?
While the facts confirm that drinking liquor can defer climax, it's anything but a treatment for untimely ejaculation.

Your urologist and group of medical care suppliers will concoct an arrangement to treat your untimely discharge. Untimely discharge is frequently effortlessly treated with a couple of basic advances, so it is essential to see your urologist or different specialists if you are encountering untimely discharge. Even with your primary care physicians about sexual issues, realize that they are experts and maintain that you and your accomplice should have a delightful sexual coexistence. Keep in mind, this is a typical issue and you are in good company!

Chapter Three

Delayed Ejaculation

Assuming that you have postponed discharge, you could start to find sexual action disappointing instead of pleasurable on account of the time allotment it takes for you to be discharged. This might be valid regardless of an accomplice. The initial step is an actual assessment

What is deferred discharge?
Deferred discharge, likewise called postponed climax, happens when you consume most of the day and need a ton of feeling to arrive at sexual peak and discharge (the term for when semen is strongly pushed out of your penis). At times, you probably won't discharge by any stretch of the imagination.

Deferred discharge, likewise called postponed climax, was recently called a male orgasmic problem. The powerlessness to discharge is called an ejaculation. Being not able to arrive at a peak (climax) is called anorgasmia.

There's no "typical" time limit for how it ought to be required to climax. Be that as it may, assuming you have deferred discharge, the time it takes might put pressure on yourself and potentially on your accomplice.

Who does deferred discharge influence?
Deferred discharge can influence anybody. It influences a few people their whole lifetime. For other people, it happens on occasion or starts to be an issue as they progress in years.

Factors that can make postponed discharge more probable include:

- Having diabetes, generally type 1 diabetes, various sclerosis, a stroke, or spinal rope injury.
- Progressing in years.

- Having had a medical procedure on your bladder or prostate.
- Taking specific meds, including a few medications that treat despondency, psychosis, hypertension, and torment.
- Psychological wellness or relationship issues.

Deferred discharge can happen while you're jerking off or while you're having intercourse with an accomplice. It very well may be something that has quite recently begun or something that has occurred all through your lifetime. If it just occurs in specific circumstances, similar to when you're with somebody, the deferred discharge could have a mental reason.

How normal is deferred discharge?
There are gauges that 1% to 4% of men in the U.S. have postponed discharge.

What are the side effects of postponed discharge?
Typically, men can discharge after just minutes of sexual excitement. One side effect of postponed discharge is that it takes you 30 minutes or more to peak.

Another issue is that you could get truly drained. You could try and begin to feel some aggravation. Both of these things could likewise be valid for your accomplice, on the off chance that there's an accomplice included. Your accomplice could feel hurt thinking they aren't adequately appealing or talented enough to invigorate you to climax.

What's significant, truly, is how you feel. On the off chance that you're baffled or resentful about the time that it takes you to discharge, or on the other hand on the off chance that you don't discharge, then, at that point, an issue should be tended to.

What causes postponed discharge?
There are physical and mental foundations for deferred discharge.

Actual causes might include:

Sensory system conditions, like stroke, spinal line injury, and numerous sclerosis. Nerve harm can likewise occur as an inconvenience of diabetes and medical procedures.

- Hypothyroidism.
- A blockage in your penis of some sort.
- Utilizing specific physician-recommended prescriptions, similar to antidepressants, or utilizing road drugs.
- Drinking liquor to overabundance.
- Maturing.
- Mental or close-to-home causes might include:
- Having a liable outlook on sex, perhaps because of your childhood.
- Feeling irate at or awkward with your accomplice.
- Fearing something, like sickness, pregnancy, or harming your accomplice.
- Having sexual execution tension.
- Being dependent on sexual entertainment.

Assuming you're ready to have a climax effectively without anyone else, yet experience issues with your accomplice, your medical services supplier could recommend that the reason isn't physical. It's likewise conceivable that you have a specific procedure that you utilize that your accomplice can't copy or that you're not happy requesting that your accomplice copy.

How is postponed discharge analyzed?
Your medical care supplier will ask you inquiries about your clinical history, sexual propensities, and discharge designs. They will preclude different circumstances, potentially doing research center testing on chemicals (testosterone), pee (pee), or semen.

At last, your sentiments about how and when you discharge are a significant piece of the finding. Your medical care supplier may likewise need to ask your accomplice a few inquiries.

How is deferred discharge treated?

Your medical services supplier might offer you various types of therapies. There truly isn't one clear method for treating the condition, however, aside from whether it's brought about by specific medications or liquor use. You can quit utilizing the medications and cut down on the drinking.

On the off chance that deferred discharges physician-recommended drugs, you can work with your medical services supplier to change to another medication that might not affect you.

Your medical care supplier could refer you to other clinical experts like a sex specialist or potentially a more conventional kind of instructor. Assuming postponed discharge happens essentially with your accomplice, your medical care supplier could recommend advising for both you and your accomplice.

If you see a sex specialist, they could propose utilizing suggestive materials or gadgets to assist you with discharging both without help from anyone else and with an accomplice.

Drugs
There is certainly not an endorsed drug treatment for deferred discharge, and that incorporates supplements. Notwithstanding, some medical services suppliers recommend medications on an "off-mark" premise with a little level of progress. A portion of these drugs are:

- Testosterone is a chemical
- Cyproheptadine (Periactin®), an allergy med.
- Buspirone (BuSpar®), is a treatment for uneasiness.
- Amantadine (Symmetrel®), is a treatment for Parkinson's infection.
- Oxytocin (Pitocin®), is a chemical utilized in labor to reinforce uterine muscle to contract and is delivered by the body during climax.
- Cabergoline is a medication that advances dopamine levels.

Remember, however, that these medications aren't intended to explicitly treat postponed discharge. They could help.

On the off chance that deferred discharge is disrupting having a youngster, your medical care supplier could recommend ways of recovering sperm that can be utilized for insemination.

Inconveniences/results of treating postponed discharge
Any medication you take can cause secondary effects. Physician-recommended drugs accompany a rundown of incidental effects to look out for.

Are there practices that will assist with deferred discharge?
You've most likely known about Kegel works out, likewise called pelvic floor works out. You can track down the muscles to practice by beginning to pee and afterward halting and beginning once more. Whenever you've found these muscles, you can do these sorts of activities in any place aipositppositionoson. It could assist you with having a more grounded pelvic floor and more command over these muscles.

How might I forestall postponed discharge?
You can't forestall postponed discharge brought about by nerve harm or maturing. You can, be that as it may, forestall issues brought about by drinking unreasonably or mishandling drugs.

On the off chance that you think relationship issues with your accomplice are considered postponed discharge, take a stab at having a fair discussion with them. Further developing your relationship might assist with keeping deferred discharge from creating or deteriorating.

What is the anticipation (standpoint) for deferred discharge?
The standpoint for deferred discharge brought about by a substance that you can stop taking is great, however, the viewpoint for postponed discharge brought about by different things isn't as great.

When would it be a good idea for me to see my medical services supplier about postponed discharge?

Assuming you've disapproved of postponed discharge, or on the other hand assuming you have fresher episodes that have endured a half year or more, call your medical care supplier. Assuming you have postponed discharge alone or with somebody and the condition is creating problems for you or your accomplice, call your medical services supplier. The primary spot to begin is to search for clinical issues that could be causing the condition, which your medical care supplier can do.

Might Viagra® at any point assist with postponed discharge?
Sildenafil (Viagra) assists individuals with erectile brokenness (ED) to last longer in sexual circumstances. It hasn't been tried in treating postponed discharge. In any case, no less than one new review showed that another ED drug, tadalafil (Cialis®), may advance discharge.

What might I do for my collaboration with postponed discharge?

Assuming you're the one conversing with your medical care supplier about deferred discharge, if it's not too much trouble, ensure your accomplice is associated with in any event a portion of the discussions. Your medical services supplier could recommend your accomplice additionally have an assessment to ensure there isn't anything physical happening with them. This is valid, particularly on the off chance that you're apprehensive about harming your accomplice during sex.

On the off chance that you're the accomplice of somebody with postponed discharge, have a go at inquiring as to whether there is something explicit you can do to help. Be available to go for couples guiding or sex treatment. In any case, attempt to relinquish the prospect that both of you are following through with something "wrong."

Deferred discharge or not discharging at everything is a condition that is as yet being contemplated. There aren't much of outright rules about how long is an excessive amount of chance to discharge, how deferred discharge ought to be dealt with or what causes it. Be that as it may, it's an issue when it's an issue for yourself and your accomplice. Many individuals could figure not being discharged for a generally significant period in a sexual circumstance would be something to be thankful for. Nonetheless, much of the time, longer sexual action isn't bringing about more joy. It's causing pressure and, surprisingly, actual issues for all accomplices included. Having fair discussions with your medical services supplier and your accomplice pretty much your concerns is all significant.

Chapter four

Retrograde Ejaculation

Retrograde discharge is additionally called dry climax. It happens when sperm doesn't leave the body through the penis but is driven once again into the bladder where pee is put away. It very well might be found during assessments.
Clinical delineation of the male regenerative framework sh the way of semen into the bladder because of retrograde discharge.
During retrograde discharge, semen enters the bladder as opposed to leaving the body through the penis.

What is retrograde discharge?

Retrograde discharge is a term that alludes to semen moving in reverse into your bladder rather than out of your body through your urethra and the tip of your penis during sexual peak. The urethra is the cylinder that lets pee and sperm leave your body.

Retrograde discharge is additionally called dry climax. It tends to be a figure of fruitlessness.

Who does retrograde discharge influence?

Retrograde discharge frequently influences people who:

- Have had a medical procedure on their prostate and urethra.
- Have diabetes or various sclerosis.
- Have harmed or had a medical procedure on their spinal strings?
- Have had pelvic or rectal medical procedures.
- Have underlying issues connected with their urethra.
- Are taking particular kinds of meds, for example, a few prostate meds, hypertension meds, or antidepressants?

How normal is retrograde discharge?
Retrograde discharge is fairly normal. For example, it occurs after most instances of transurethral resection of the prostate (TURP) medical procedures. TURP is utilized to treat harmless prostatic hyperplasia, additionally called a broadened prostate.

Conditions that might cause retrograde discharge are additionally fairly normal, like diabetes. As far as meds, people who consume medications for hypertension or sorrow might foster retrograde discharge.

What are the signs and side effects of retrograde discharge?
You probably won't see on the off chance that you have retrograde discharge. On the other hand, you can see the following:

- You produce next to zero semen when you climax.
- You have shady pee after you climax.
- You're having fruitfulness issues.

What causes retrograde discharge?
Retrograde discharge is brought about by an issue with your round muscle (called the bladder sphincter) that closes to let semen out and keeps pee in your body. Since your sphincter doesn't work accurately, your bladder neck stays open as opposed to shutting permitting the discharge to follow the easy way out into the bladder.

How is retrograde discharge analyzed?
Your supplier will ask you inquiries about your side effects and will do an actual assessment. Then, at that point, to analyze retrograde discharge, your medical care supplier might request that you give:

Semen tests. If you produce an exceptionally low volume of semen in something like two examples, you could have retrograde discharge.

A pee test is taken just after you climax. Fructose is available in semen tests. If you have retrograde discharge, research center tests will track down fructose in your pee. The lab will likewise break down the quantity of sperm in your pee.

How is retrograde discharge treated?
Retrograde discharge doesn't appear to be agonizing or unsafe. If you don't need kids, your supplier might propose that it doesn't require treatment.

Nonetheless, assuming you conclude you need treatment, some prescriptions assist the sphincter with shutting firmly. These incorporate imipramine, a more seasoned energizer, and allergy meds like pseudoephedrine and chlorpheniramine.

If your condition is being brought about by the meds you're on, talk with your supplier about rolling out an improvement to an alternate kind of medication.

What are a few difficulties or incidental effects connected with drug treatment of retrograde discharge?
Assuming you have retrograde discharge and you take imipramine or pseudoephedrine, your medical care supplier will watch out for your pulse and pulse. The medications increment both circulatory strain and pulse.

On the off chance that the medications don't attempt to assist with retrograde discharge, there are still ways of helping fruitfulness. For example, your supplier can gather your sperm with the goal that it tends to be utilized for insemination.

Are there practices that assist with retretrograde mightn't know which ones these are by halting and beginning yoyou're m while .o?mwhileu're g. Practicing them includes crushing and delivering these muscles. These activities are frequently called Kegel works.

How might I forestall retrograde discharge?

It's impossible to forestall retrograde discharge. However, assuming you have diabetes, it's vital to keep your glucose levels consistent. It's crucial for your general well-being as well as your peni's well-being.

What is the viewpoint (guess) for retrograde discharge?
Medical care experts don't completely accept that retrograde discharge is unsafe or agonizing. Your standpoint is great, except if you're attempting to have youngsters. And still, after all that, there are medicines for both retrograde discharge and barrenness.

When would it be advisable for me to see my medical care supplier regarding retrograde?
You need to contact your medical care supplier if:

- You're attempting to have kids and things aren't advancing.
- You're awkward with how things feel when you climax.
- You're being treated for retrograde discharge, and treatment isn't working.

What in all actuality does retrograde discharge feel like?
Retrograde discharge feels equivalent to antegrade discharge. Antegrade discharge is the term for semen strongly being pushed out of the body through the penis, instead of being powerfully driven once again into the bladder. Nonetheless, if you're awkward under any condition with the absence of semen during the climax, contact your medical care supplier.

Does retrograde discharge disappear?
Retrograde discharge can disappear with treatment. It can likewise disappear assuming you're ready to change the drugs that cause it.

How normal is retrograde discharge after transurethral resection of the prostate (TURP)?
The pace of retrograde discharge after TURP is assessed to be essentially as high as 70% to 90%. If the bladder neck is saved during TURP, there might be less gamble of retrograde discharge.

Are there advantages to retrograde discharge?

Certain individuals accept that holding sperm will expand their testosterone levels or will permit them to live longer. These individuals try to prevent themselves from discharging outside the body. Nonetheless, this is dubious and not suggested by most medical care suppliers.

Retrograde discharge is a fairly normal event because of many causes, including prescription use, medical procedures, and ailments. While medical care suppliers don't view it as being difficult or destructive, it very well may be an issue for individuals who need to consider it. There are ways of treating retrograde discharge. Address your medical care supplier about any of your interests.